# The OCD Recovery Journal

# The OCD Recovery Journal

## Creative Activities to Keep Yourself Well

### CARA LISETTE and PHOEBE WEBB

Foreword by Ashley Fulwood
Illustrated by Victoria Barron

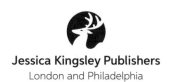

**Jessica Kingsley Publishers**
London and Philadelphia

First published in Great Britain in 2024 by Jessica Kingsley Publishers
An imprint of John Murray Press

1

A CIP catalogue record for this title is available from the
British Library and the Library of Congress

ISBN 978 1 80501 095 1
eISBN 978 1 80501 096 8

Printed and bound in Great Britain by Bell & Bain Limited

Jessica Kingsley Publishers' policy is to use papers that are natural, renewable and recyclable
products and made from wood grown in sustainable forests. The logging and manufacturing
processes are expected to conform to the environmental regulations of the country of origin.

Jessica Kingsley Publishers
Carmelite House
50 Victoria Embankment
London EC4Y 0DZ

www.jkp.com

John Murray Press
Part of Hodder & Stoughton Ltd
An Hachette Company

# Foreword

Being asked to write a foreword for a book is always an honour, but even more so when the authors are people who've experienced OCD or mental health problems themselves. Throughout this book Cara and Phoebe's own experiences are evident as they write with such compassion and determination to help the reader move forward in their journey.

Whilst reviewing the book for this foreword I found myself constantly reading out extracts to my colleagues here at OCD-UK and exclaiming how much I love what Cara and Phoebe had written, and I am sure you, the reader, will be equally inspired.

If I was to be honest, I would say that a creative journal is not the kind of book I would normally pick up, but within those first inspiring pages I was not only encouraged to keep reading, but convinced this was a book I would recommend to anyone who is suffering from obsessive-compulsive disorder, and a book I would be honoured to write a foreword for.

Through this book the reader is taken on a journey of helping us identify the resources we need to work towards our own individual recovery and to create our own toolkit of recovery resources. Readers are invited to write or let their creative juices flow with practical and cathartic written or creative exercises.

Cara expresses the desire and wish that they have created a resource that will be helpful for readers whatever stage of their journey they are at, and I can assure her that they have done just that! Not only would this journal have helped me at the start of my OCD journey living with and tackling this insidious condition, it has also helped me today as someone working towards complete recovery from OCD. As Cara and Phoebe write, *recovery is a direction*, and this book is a wonderful resource to help you stay on course.

That's not to say they have done all the work for you by writing this book, but what they have done is created a journal for you to express yourself in writing or using creativity should you wish to.

How much you get from this book could be determined by how much you use it as intended. It forces us to think hard about our OCD and the impact on our lives, and what we can do to move ourselves forward. I know only too well from my own therapeutic experiences just how challenging, but necessary, that level of deep thinking and appraisal can be at times; however, Cara and Phoebe have written this in a way that is supportive and compassionate to help us work towards achieving our recovery and life goals.

Having such goals is an often overlooked aspect of therapy, but when therapy gets tough, and it does, having such goals can keep us grounded and motivated to keep working through the challenges of OCD.

Make no mistake, this is a book about OCD recovery and written with compassion from the authors and ensuring that we can use our own self-compassion at the forefront of the journal. As Cara and Phoebe write, *'there is more to you than OCD, and...you can make positive steps to living a full and happy life.'* This journal can be another fantastic resource to help you along that journey.

This is a wonderful book that will be both practical and comforting when living with and working towards recovery from obsessive-compulsive disorder.

*Ashley Fulwood*
*Chief Executive of the national charity OCD-UK*
*and someone with lived experience of OCD*

Hello, reader!

Welcome to this journal, which we hope you will be able to use to learn more about yourself and your experiences of OCD. Throughout this book there are a number of exercises to help you to explore different coping strategies, and ideas to help you to start challenging your OCD.

We have used our knowledge, through both Cara's clinical and personal experiences as a trained therapist with mental health difficulties and Phoebe's lived experience of OCD and peer support work, to provide evidence-based techniques and exercises designed to help you to tap into your creative side and take control of your OCD.

It was important to us when putting the journal together that we had input from somebody who has experienced living with OCD and all the various challenges that come along with this diagnosis. Though most of the evidence-based techniques come from Cara's training as a mental health nurse and therapist, Phoebe, who has lived with OCD for a long time, has contributed huge amounts to some of the more creative activities.

This is your book to use as you choose: you can write in it, draw in it, decorate it - creativity is an excellent outlet and our aim is that you find that some of these prompts bring you closer to where you want to be.

This journal is not a replacement for therapy, but a tool to help you to learn more about your OCD and different strategies that may help you to make changes that have a positive impact on your life.

Never forget that there is more to you than OCD, and that you can make positive steps to living a full and happy life.

Lots of love, Cara and Phoebe

## A note from Phoebe

Hello! I'm Phoebe and I have OCD, and that is the least inter-esting thing about me. I admit that I didn't always believe that; I thought OCD was the ONLY thing about me. OCD and I have known each other for about 20 years, and it has taken many forms in that time. You could say it's a love/hate relationship. After all this time, though, our relationship is starting to fizzle and I'm ready to move on. I've contributed to this book as some-one going through recovery in real time, so I could be feeling similarly to how you feel right now. Scared, angry, bored, even? Let's feel that. Let's use that. This is our rocket fuel for change, change that we deserve. I see the power of lived experience and peer support every day in my work, and hope to spread that even further through this recovery journal.

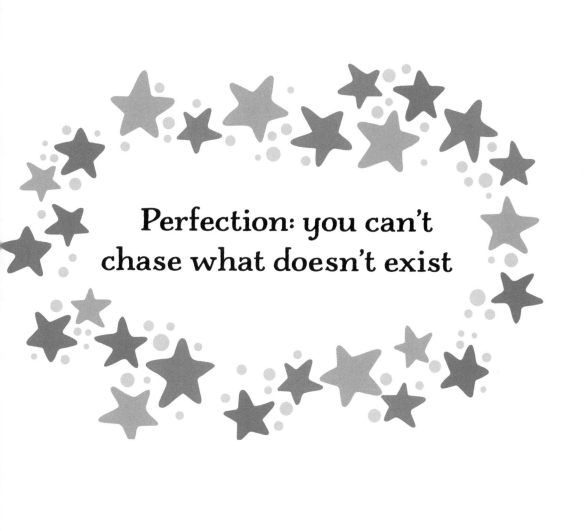

Perfection: you can't
chase what doesn't exist

# What is OCD?

Obsessive-compulsive disorder (OCD) is a mental illness that can be broken down into two parts: obsessions, which are intrusive thoughts, images or impulses, and compulsions, which are repetitive physical or mental behaviours which are difficult to stop. People who live with OCD experience high levels of anxiety that can have a significant impact on their day-to-day functioning.

OCD affects people of all ages, races and genders, and everyone's experience of it will be unique – no two presentations of OCD are the same and there are lots of different obsessions and compulsions that people might experience.

When we think of OCD, an image is often conjured up of somebody who washes their hands a lot or who lines up their books neatly. Whilst it is true that some people with OCD will experience fears around contamination or a need for things to be orderly, this is a stereotype that does not capture all the many different ways OCD can present. Many parts of OCD are often unspoken, such as strong fears people may have that they are going to harm themselves or somebody else, and though this doesn't mean they are likely to actually do this, they may go to extreme lengths to prevent this from happening due to the high levels of distress these thoughts can cause. Due to the secretive nature of these types of thoughts, lots of people with OCD may not realize that they have it, and can go years without the right treatment and support.

It is important to recognize that even if your symptoms don't match the OCD stereotype, you still deserve help and support, and your difficulties are just as valid.

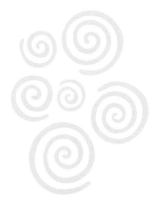

# My goals for the future

Start by setting yourself some goals. What would you like to achieve, and by when? It is important to set goals that feel realistic. Most people will experience intrusive thoughts from time to time, so perhaps a goal might be not to get rid of them entirely but to reduce the anxiety associated with them. It can also be helpful to focus on ways you would like your life to be different, or things you'd like to be doing more or less of.

1. ..................................................................................................
..................................................................................................

2. ..................................................................................................
..................................................................................................

3. ..................................................................................................
..................................................................................................

4. ..................................................................................................
..................................................................................................

5. ..................................................................................................
..................................................................................................

6. ..................................................................................................
..................................................................................................

7. ..................................................................................................
..................................................................................................

8. ..................................................................................................
..................................................................................................

9. ..................................................................................................
..................................................................................................

10. ..................................................................................................
..................................................................................................

# My reasons to recover

1. .............................................................................................
.............................................................................................

2. .............................................................................................
.............................................................................................

3. .............................................................................................
.............................................................................................

4. .............................................................................................
.............................................................................................

5. .............................................................................................
.............................................................................................

6. .............................................................................................
.............................................................................................

7. .............................................................................................
.............................................................................................

8. .............................................................................................
.............................................................................................

9. .............................................................................................
.............................................................................................

10. .............................................................................................
.............................................................................................

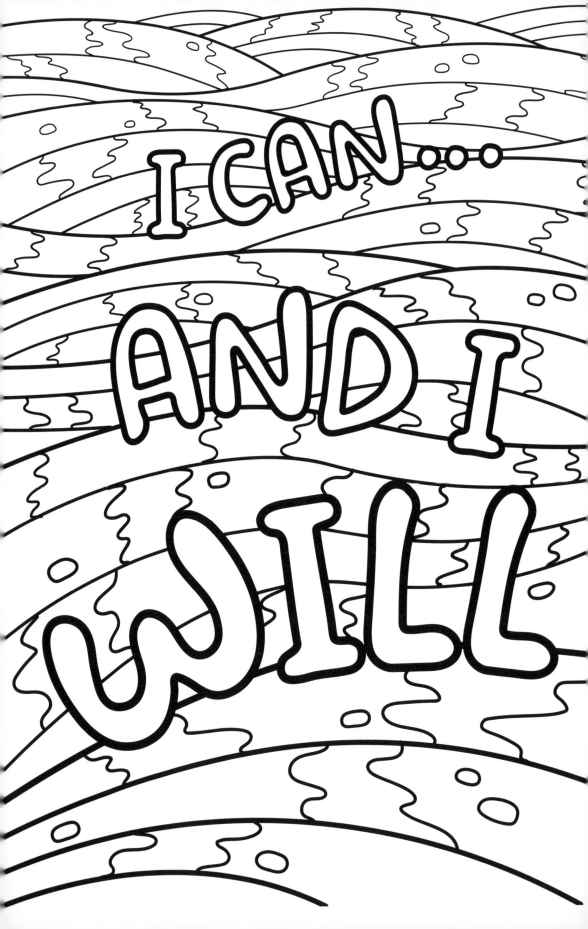

# Brain dump

How are you feeling right now? Sometimes getting our thoughts out onto the page can help us to process and make sense of them.

..............................................................................

..............................................................................

..............................................................................

..............................................................................

..............................................................................

..............................................................................

..............................................................................

..............................................................................

..............................................................................

..............................................................................

..............................................................................

..............................................................................

..............................................................................

..............................................................................

..............................................................................

..............................................................................

..............................................................................

..............................................................................

# What does my life look like with OCD?

OCD can take up huge amounts of time and energy, and can ultimately get in the way of a lot of other things in our life that are important to us. Think of this circle as being your life right now. If you were to divide it into a pie chart, how much of that would be OCD, and how much would be left for everything else – work, friends, hobbies? For example, maybe OCD is taking up 80% of your energy and thoughts right now. Doing this exercise can help motivate us to make changes, so that the pie chart of our lives can be full of the things we care about and value.

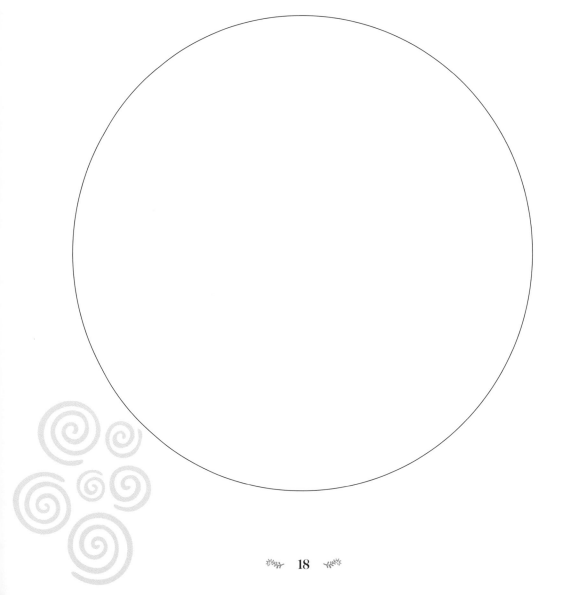

# What does a day look like with OCD?

Now that we've had a think about how your life overall is structured, let's think about what a typical day looks like for you right now, focusing on not just your OCD thoughts and behaviours, but other things you do too.

# What does my life look like without OCD?

Now think about what the pie chart of your life would look like if OCD wasn't there. How much time would you like to dedicate to things you enjoy? Perhaps you'd like to spend a quarter of your life at work, and a lot more of it socializing. Maybe you love studying and want to spend a third of your time doing that. If travelling is your goal, it might take up most of your circle. This is your individual pie chart, and should align with your own goals and values.

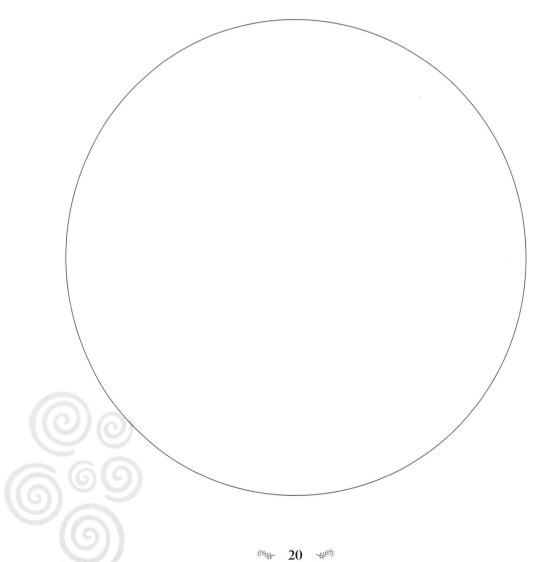

# What does a day look like without OCD?

Now that we've had a think about how you'd like to spend your time in an ideal world, let's have a think about what a typical day would be like for you if your OCD was gone or less present than it is right now.

# Helpful mantras

I am much more than my thoughts

There is life beyond the confounds of OCD

I am worthy of a full life

Feel the fear and do it anyway

Become the person you've always needed

My demons are strong, but I am stronger

Every emotion serves a purpose

To struggle is not to discount progress

I am proud of myself for trying

Recovery is not a big decision. It is a series of tiny decisions

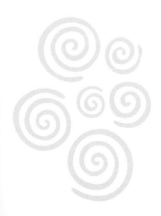

# Activities that help me to get out of my head

OCD can make our lives feel small, and connecting to things we enjoy can be a good motivator and help us reconnect with ourselves.

There are some suggestions here that might help, but you will probably have some of your own too.

- ❀ Writing
- ❀ Drawing
- ❀ Reading a book
- ❀ Watching a film
- ❀ Listening to podcasts or a happy playlist
- ❀ Arts and crafts
- ❀ Painting your nails
- ❀ Having a bath or shower
- ❀ Crossword puzzles
- ❀ Playing a game
- ❀ Colouring books

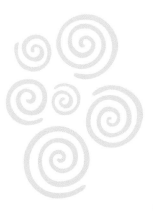

# Activities that help me

You might already have your own ideas for activities that you enjoy. Write down some ideas that you could try if you need to take your mind off things.

1. ........................................................................................
   ........................................................................................

2. ........................................................................................
   ........................................................................................

3. ........................................................................................
   ........................................................................................

4. ........................................................................................
   ........................................................................................

5. ........................................................................................
   ........................................................................................

6. ........................................................................................
   ........................................................................................

7. ........................................................................................
   ........................................................................................

8. ........................................................................................
   ........................................................................................

9. ........................................................................................
   ........................................................................................

10. ........................................................................................
    ........................................................................................

**How are you feeling today? Draw or write it out!**

# My support network

It's important to reach out for help when we are struggling, whether that be to friends, family, mental health professionals or charities, for example. Have a think about who is in your network and who you can reach out to when you need support.

## Friends:

.................................................................................

.................................................................................

.................................................................................

.................................................................................

.................................................................................

.................................................................................

## Family:

.................................................................................

.................................................................................

.................................................................................

.................................................................................

.................................................................................

.................................................................................

## Professionals:

. . . . . . . . . . . . . . . . . . . . . . . . . . . . . . . . . . . . . . . . . . . . . . . . . . . . . . . . . . . . . . . . . . . . . . . . . .

. . . . . . . . . . . . . . . . . . . . . . . . . . . . . . . . . . . . . . . . . . . . . . . . . . . . . . . . . . . . . . . . . . . . . . . . . .

. . . . . . . . . . . . . . . . . . . . . . . . . . . . . . . . . . . . . . . . . . . . . . . . . . . . . . . . . . . . . . . . . . . . . . . . . .

. . . . . . . . . . . . . . . . . . . . . . . . . . . . . . . . . . . . . . . . . . . . . . . . . . . . . . . . . . . . . . . . . . . . . . . . . .

. . . . . . . . . . . . . . . . . . . . . . . . . . . . . . . . . . . . . . . . . . . . . . . . . . . . . . . . . . . . . . . . . . . . . . . . . .

. . . . . . . . . . . . . . . . . . . . . . . . . . . . . . . . . . . . . . . . . . . . . . . . . . . . . . . . . . . . . . . . . . . . . . . . . .

## Other:

. . . . . . . . . . . . . . . . . . . . . . . . . . . . . . . . . . . . . . . . . . . . . . . . . . . . . . . . . . . . . . . . . . . . . . . . . .

. . . . . . . . . . . . . . . . . . . . . . . . . . . . . . . . . . . . . . . . . . . . . . . . . . . . . . . . . . . . . . . . . . . . . . . . . .

. . . . . . . . . . . . . . . . . . . . . . . . . . . . . . . . . . . . . . . . . . . . . . . . . . . . . . . . . . . . . . . . . . . . . . . . . .

. . . . . . . . . . . . . . . . . . . . . . . . . . . . . . . . . . . . . . . . . . . . . . . . . . . . . . . . . . . . . . . . . . . . . . . . . .

. . . . . . . . . . . . . . . . . . . . . . . . . . . . . . . . . . . . . . . . . . . . . . . . . . . . . . . . . . . . . . . . . . . . . . . . . .

. . . . . . . . . . . . . . . . . . . . . . . . . . . . . . . . . . . . . . . . . . . . . . . . . . . . . . . . . . . . . . . . . . . . . . . . . .

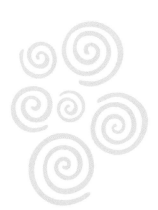

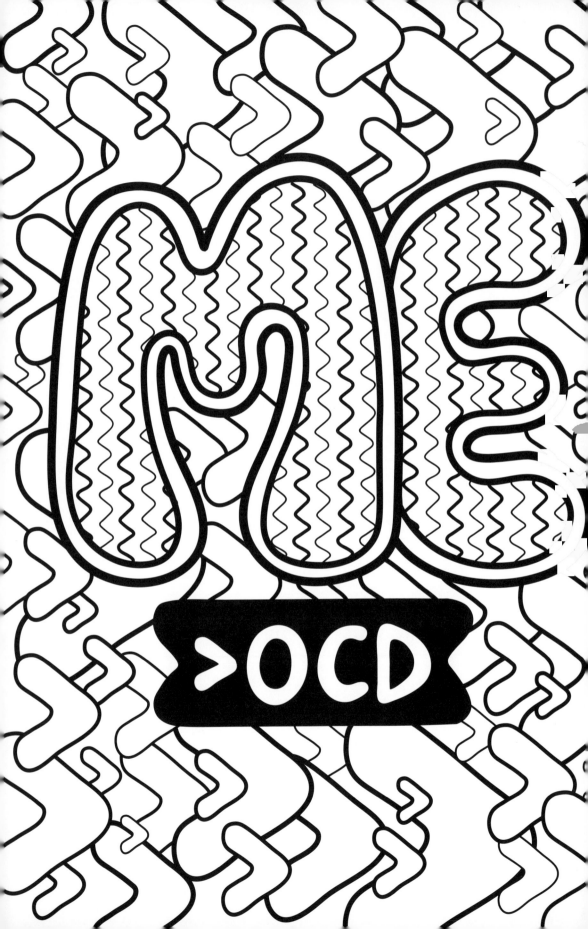

# What is important to me?

When we are struggling with our mental health it can be really difficult to remember what is important to us. Try and make a list of things that are important to you.

1. ......................................................................

......................................................................

2. ......................................................................

......................................................................

3. ......................................................................

......................................................................

4. ......................................................................

......................................................................

5. ......................................................................

......................................................................

6. ......................................................................

......................................................................

7. ......................................................................

......................................................................

8. ......................................................................

......................................................................

9. ......................................................................

......................................................................

10. ......................................................................

......................................................................

# What are my values?

Our values are what guide the way we behave, both towards others and towards ourselves. It can be useful to identify our values as this can help us to establish changes we want to make, so we can align our actions closer to the things that are important to us. Here is a list of values that you might connect with. It might help to highlight some, but there is also space to record your own that don't feature here.

| | | |
|---|---|---|
| Achievement | Growth | Optimism |
| Adventure | Hope | Peace |
| Braveness | Independence | Productivity |
| Community | Individuality | Quality |
| Compassion | Intelligence | Recreation |
| Connection | Joy | Reflection |
| Dedication | Justice | Security |
| Discovery | Kindness | Spirituality |
| Empowerment | Knowledge | Success |
| Equality | Learning | Teamwork |
| Family | Love | Tolerance |
| Freedom | Motivation | Truthfulness |
| Fun | Nourishment | Unity |
| Generosity | Nurture | Wealth |

........................     ........................     ........................
........................     ........................     ........................
........................     ........................     ........................
........................     ........................     ........................
........................     ........................     ........................
........................     ........................     ........................
........................     ........................     ........................
........................     ........................     ........................

## What changes can I make that will bring me closer to living a life aligned with my values?

Are there any moves you can make to move closer to your values, such as your relationships, career, education or hobbies?

.......................................................................

.......................................................................

.......................................................................

.......................................................................

.......................................................................

.......................................................................

.......................................................................

.......................................................................

.......................................................................

.......................................................................

.......................................................................

.......................................................................

.......................................................................

.......................................................................

.......................................................................

.......................................................................

.......................................................................

.......................................................................

.......................................................................

# Brain dump

How are you feeling right now? Sometimes getting our thoughts out onto the page can help us to process and make sense of them.

..........................................................................................

..........................................................................................

..........................................................................................

..........................................................................................

..........................................................................................

..........................................................................................

..........................................................................................

..........................................................................................

..........................................................................................

..........................................................................................

..........................................................................................

..........................................................................................

..........................................................................................

..........................................................................................

..........................................................................................

..........................................................................................

..........................................................................................

..........................................................................................

# Signs I am feeling anxious

How do you know when you are feeling anxious? What physical sensations or feelings might you notice? What behaviours might those around you see?

..........................................................................................

..........................................................................................

..........................................................................................

..........................................................................................

..........................................................................................

..........................................................................................

..........................................................................................

..........................................................................................

..........................................................................................

..........................................................................................

..........................................................................................

..........................................................................................

..........................................................................................

..........................................................................................

..........................................................................................

..........................................................................................

..........................................................................................

..........................................................................................

..........................................................................................

..........................................................................................

# Drawing emotions

As we may have noticed in the previous page, emotions are physical! On the gingerbread person below add colours or words to represent how your body feels when you are anxious. Is your chest tight? Do you feel dizzy? Connect with your body and consider what you could do to manage those symptoms – you might even find some strategies you haven't thought of as you work your way through this book.

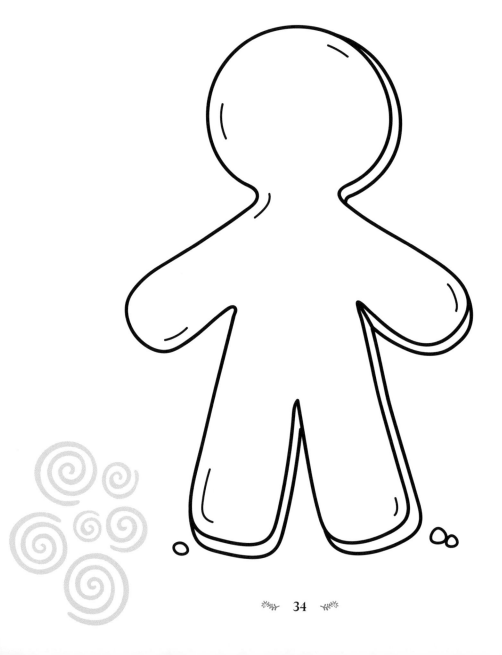

# What healthy coping strategies can I use when I am feeling anxious?

# How can other people help me when I am feeling anxious?

# What does OCD look like to you?

It can be really helpful when trying to challenge OCD to think of it as something separate from us. What does your OCD look like, and what does it say to you?

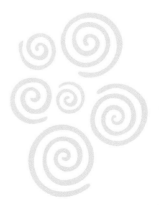

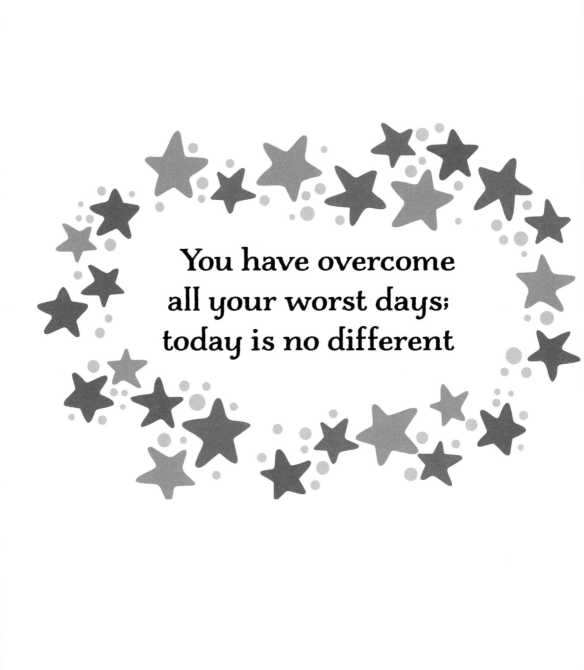

You have overcome
all your worst days;
today is no different

# How are you feeling today? Draw or write it out!

# OCD diary

Keeping an OCD diary can be really helpful in helping us to really notice patterns in our thoughts, feelings and behaviours, and what might be triggering them. Use the template below to get you started.

| Time/date | What was happening? | How was I feeling? |
|---|---|---|
| | | |
| | | |
| | | |
| | | |
| | | |
| | | |
| | | |
| | | |
| | | |
| | | |

| What were my intrusive thoughts? | What compulsions did I do? |
| --- | --- |
|  |  |
|  |  |
|  |  |
|  |  |
|  |  |
|  |  |
|  |  |
|  |  |
|  |  |
|  |  |
|  |  |

# OCD cycle

We can think of OCD as being like a cycle. We experience an intrusive thought, image or urge (obsession), become anxious, and do something to reduce this anxiety (compulsion). This works temporarily by relieving anxiety but ultimately reinforces the cycle. So the next time an obsession arises, we do the compulsion again. However, as I am sure you will know if you are reading this, the relief from doing the compulsion is short lived and the obsession returns, often bigger and stronger. This leads to people having to carry out more and more compulsions to relieve anxiety and becoming stuck in the obsession/compulsion loop.

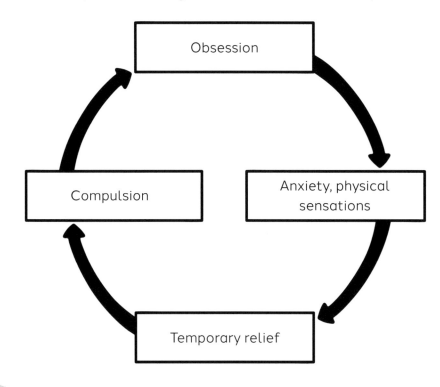

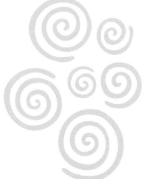

# OCD hot cross buns

As we can see in the OCD cycle, our thoughts, feelings and behaviours all connect to one another. The way we behave can affect how we think and feel, and trying to change our thinking can impact what we do and what emotions we are experiencing. A 'hot cross bun' is a cognitive behavioural therapy diagram that shows us how our thoughts, feelings, physical sensations and behaviours are all interconnected.

For example, if you heard a sudden noise in the middle of the night you might have different thoughts about what it is, which would influence the way you feel and how you respond. Have a go at writing two different thoughts you might have about the noise (e.g. was it a burglar, was it a cat?) and the different feelings and behaviours you would experience as a result of each different thought.

## A noise in the night

You hear a noise in the night and you think it might be something scary…

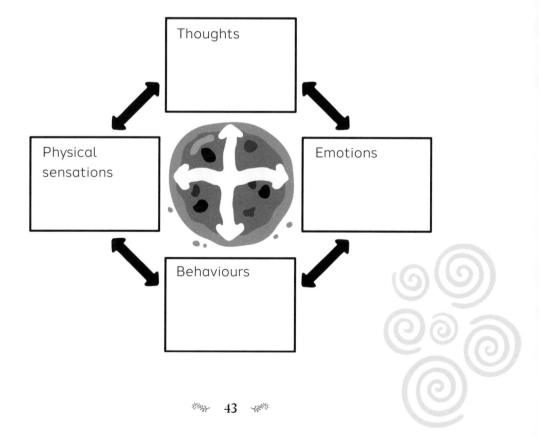

When we experience scary thoughts, we are more likely to feel anxious.
We can try challenging these thoughts by coming up with alternative,
less threatening thoughts, which impact on how we feel and behave.
Can you come up with a less scary thought about the noise in the night?
How would this change the cycle?

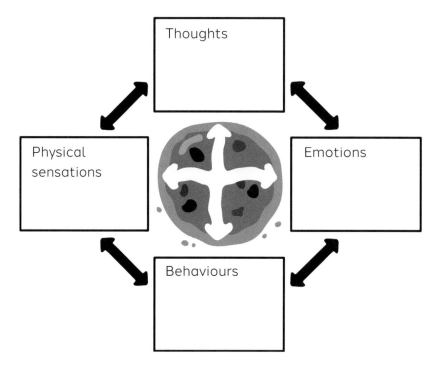

Thoughts

Physical sensations

Emotions

Behaviours

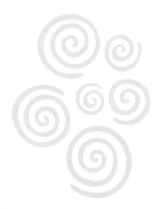

Now try mapping out your own hot cross bun with an experience you have as a result of OCD. What are your current thoughts, feelings, behaviours and physical sensations?

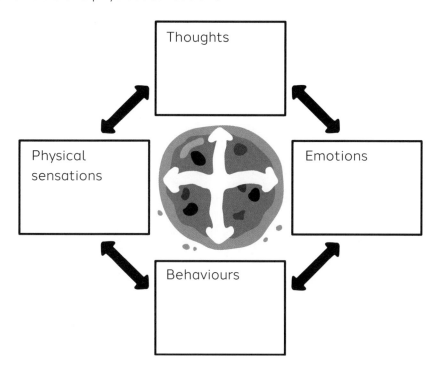

Now try to imagine an alternative example. Are there any other ways you could respond to the obsessions or any ways you could challenge these thoughts? What impact would that have on how you feel?

..................................................................................

..................................................................................

..................................................................................

..................................................................................

..................................................................................

..................................................................................

..................................................................................

..................................................................................

..................................................................................

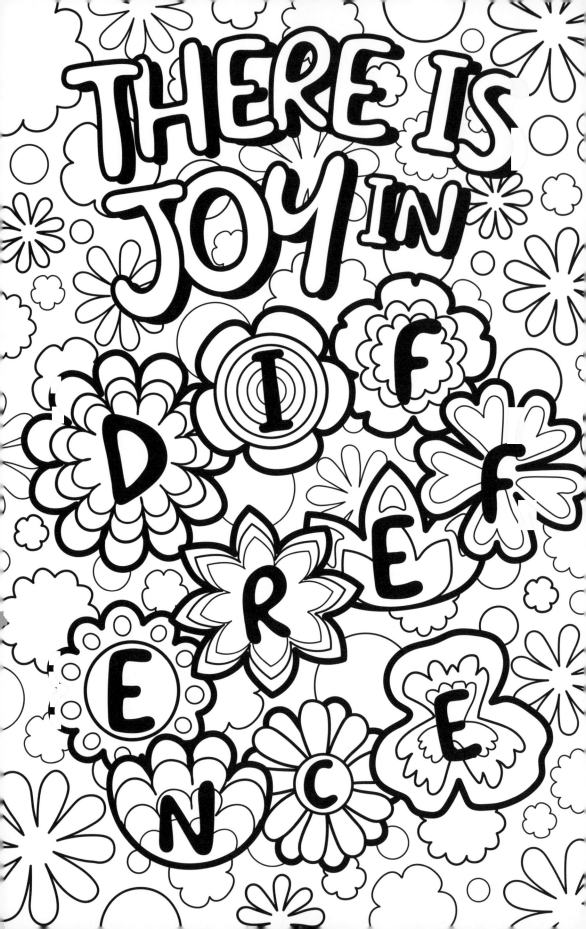

# Brain dump

How are you feeling right now? Sometimes getting our thoughts out onto the page can help us to process and make sense of them.

.................................................................................

.................................................................................

.................................................................................

.................................................................................

.................................................................................

.................................................................................

.................................................................................

.................................................................................

.................................................................................

.................................................................................

.................................................................................

.................................................................................

.................................................................................

.................................................................................

.................................................................................

.................................................................................

.................................................................................

.................................................................................

.................................................................................

.................................................................................

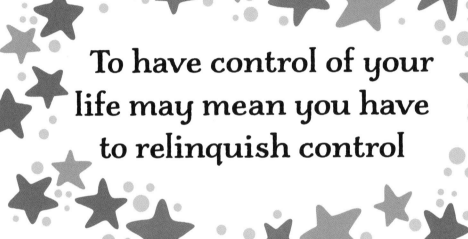

To have control of your life may mean you have to relinquish control

# Collage making

Thoughts and emotions can be hard to put into words. Try creating a collage from newspapers, magazines, household objects, greetings cards and more to make a visual representation of what you are experiencing. This might also be a helpful way to communicate how you are feeling with others, if you're finding it difficult to talk.

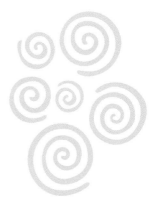

# Letter writing

Intrusive thoughts can be completely all consuming and feel impossible to ignore at times. What would you like to say to yourself next time you are experiencing intrusive thoughts? How can you be kind and compassionate to yourself?

..................................................................................
..................................................................................
..................................................................................
..................................................................................
..................................................................................
..................................................................................
..................................................................................
..................................................................................
..................................................................................

Compulsions can feel very difficult to stop and it's easy to feel stuck and overwhelmed when you're caught up in them. What would you like to say to yourself next time you're struggling with compulsions?

..................................................................................
..................................................................................
..................................................................................
..................................................................................
..................................................................................
..................................................................................
..................................................................................
..................................................................................

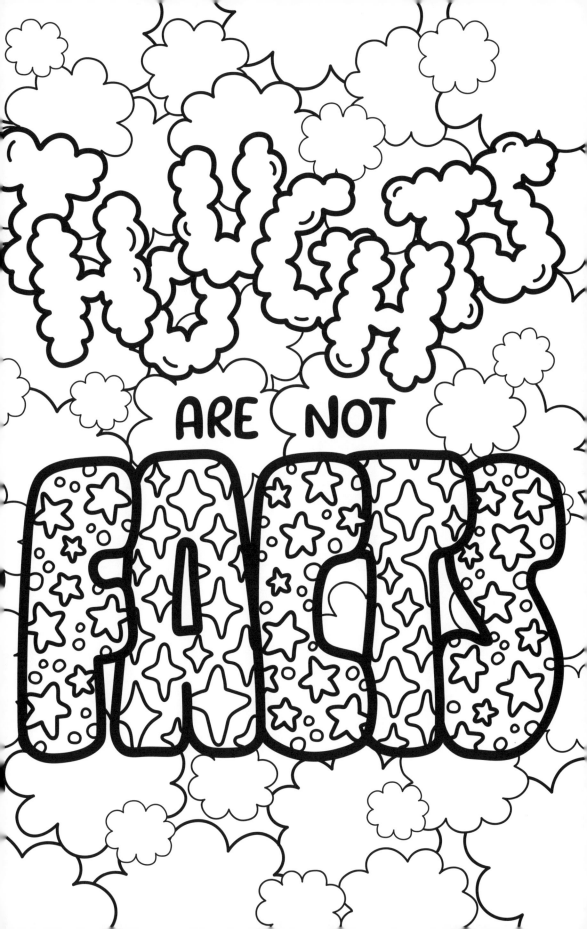

# Taking back control

When OCD takes hold, it can feel like it's controlling everything you think and do. Sometimes it can help to put this in perspective by recognizing areas in which we do still have control over our lives. Let's think about some areas where OCD does currently have complete control, some where it has a little bit, and times where you have total control. Once you get to the end of this journal, it might be useful to reflect back on this exercise to see if there are any areas where OCD used to be in total control but you managed to regain some or all of it back.

## What is OCD currently in control of?

..................................................................................................

..................................................................................................

..................................................................................................

..................................................................................................

..................................................................................................

..................................................................................................

..................................................................................................

..................................................................................................

..................................................................................................

## What does OCD sometimes control?

...............................................................

...............................................................

...............................................................

...............................................................

...............................................................

...............................................................

...............................................................

...............................................................

...............................................................

## What am I in control of?

...............................................................

...............................................................

...............................................................

...............................................................

...............................................................

...............................................................

...............................................................

...............................................................

...............................................................

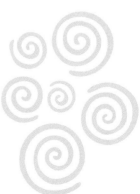

# How are you feeling today? Draw or write it out!

# Miracle question

If you were to wake up tomorrow and your OCD was gone, what would life look like?

..................................................................
..................................................................
..................................................................
..................................................................
..................................................................
..................................................................
..................................................................
..................................................................
..................................................................
..................................................................
..................................................................
..................................................................
..................................................................
..................................................................
..................................................................
..................................................................
..................................................................
..................................................................
..................................................................
..................................................................

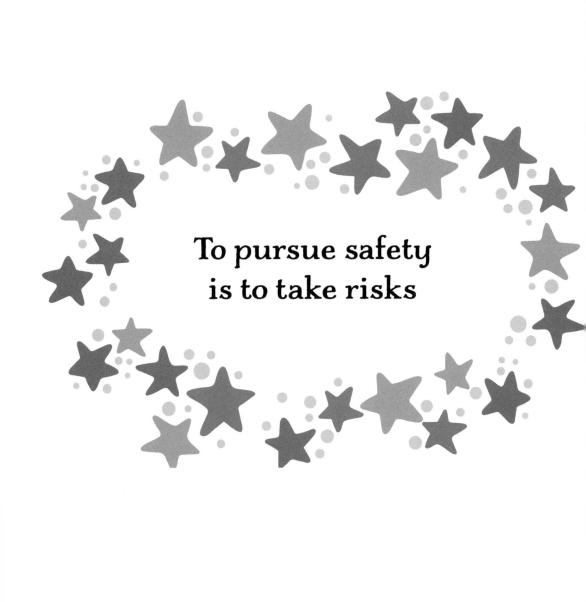

To pursue safety
is to take risks

# Self-care activities

It can feel difficult to look after ourselves when we are struggling with our mental health. One of the best ways to challenge this is to start being kind to ourselves. What self-care activities can you try?

1. ............................................................................
............................................................................

2. ............................................................................
............................................................................

3. ............................................................................
............................................................................

4. ............................................................................
............................................................................

5. ............................................................................
............................................................................

6. ............................................................................
............................................................................

7. ............................................................................
............................................................................

8. ............................................................................
............................................................................

9. ............................................................................
............................................................................

10. ............................................................................
............................................................................

# 31 days of self-care

| | | |
|---|---|---|
| **1**<br>Unfollow unhelpful pages on social media | **2**<br>Identify five things you are grateful for today | **3**<br>Learn self-massage techniques |
| **8**<br>Start the day with your favourite breakfast | **9**<br>Try a new recipe | **10**<br>Engage with something that makes you laugh |
| **15**<br>Check out good news websites | **16**<br>Keep hydrated | **17**<br>Check in with your body throughout the day |
| **22**<br>Take an hour of no screen time | **23**<br>Wear your comfiest clothes | **24**<br>Wear clothes that make you feel like a boss |
| **29**<br>Make a new happy playlist | **30**<br>Have some screen-free time before you go to sleep | **31**<br>Have an uninterrupted comforting hot drink |

| | | | |
|---|---|---|---|
| 4<br>Search for images of your favourite animal | 5<br>Listen to a new podcast or YouTube channel | 6<br>Say aloud three things you appreciate about yourself | 7<br>Move your body in a way that feels good |
| 11<br>Listen to an empowering song | 12<br>Take photos of five things that make you feel good | 13<br>Try a word puzzle or sudoku | 14<br>Contact someone you haven't spoken to in a while |
| 18<br>Talk to yourself how you would a friend | 19<br>Try a new hobby and allow yourself to not be good at it | 20<br>Spend some time outdoors | 21<br>Build a fort and embrace your inner child |
| 25<br>Rewatch your comfort show/film | 26<br>Spend five minutes stretching | 27<br>Eat what you're craving | 28<br>Ask for help with something |
| | | | |

# Brain dump

How are you feeling right now? Sometimes getting our thoughts out onto the page can help us to process and make sense of them.

........................................................................

........................................................................

........................................................................

........................................................................

........................................................................

........................................................................

........................................................................

........................................................................

........................................................................

........................................................................

........................................................................

........................................................................

........................................................................

........................................................................

........................................................................

........................................................................

........................................................................

........................................................................

# How are you feeling today? Draw or write it out!

# Quotes, lyrics and phrases that inspire me

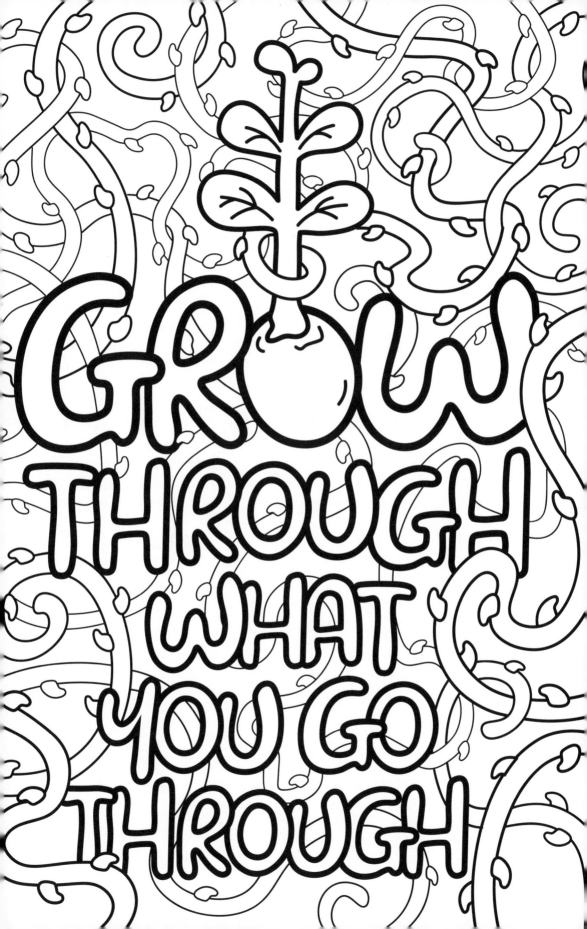

# 54321 grounding technique

Anxiety and distress can feel completely overwhelming sometimes. If you find yourself feeling like this, this technique can be very effective at bringing you back into the here and now by helping you to connect to your senses. There are five steps to follow.

1. Look around you and notice **five things you can see**. This could be a painting, a plant or a person, for example. Pay attention to what each of these things look like: their shapes, colours and sizes.

2. Focus on **four things you can feel**. This could be the wind, your clothes against your skin, the floor underneath your feet. Notice the different textures and sensations.

3. Name **three things you can hear**. Maybe there are birds chirping outside, or cars passing in the street. Perhaps you can hear a TV show in the background. Focus on the different tones and volumes.

4. Notice **two things you can smell**. Have you used a nice fabric softener on your clothes, or are you wearing your favourite perfume? Maybe you are outdoors and can smell plants and flowers.

5. Think about **one thing you can taste**. Perhaps you have chewing gum or a cup of tea nearby. If you can't taste anything, try to imagine what one of your favourite things tastes like.

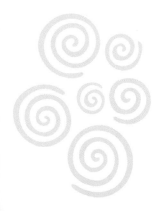

# The power of music

Music can be an amazing tool for our wellbeing, and there are so many inspiring songs and artists out there. What songs give you inspiration and motivation?

....................................................................................

....................................................................................

....................................................................................

....................................................................................

....................................................................................

....................................................................................

....................................................................................

....................................................................................

....................................................................................

....................................................................................

....................................................................................

....................................................................................

....................................................................................

....................................................................................

....................................................................................

....................................................................................

....................................................................................

....................................................................................

....................................................................................

....................................................................................

# Square breathing technique

Square breathing has been shown to be helpful when trying to relax and feel calm, and is an exercise that can be used wherever you are. Find a window, a wall, a painting or any other square shape you can see to focus on. If you can't see one, you can use your index finger to trace one in front of you.

Slowly trace your eyes across the top of the square in front of you, breathing in for a count of four. As you scan down the right side of the square, hold your breath for a count of four. Breathe out for a count of four as you trace the bottom of the square, then hold for a count of four as you scan up the left hand side. Repeat this as many times as necessary, breathing in a slow and controlled way.

It is important when directly challenging OCD that we try to focus on what the task is at hand. However, square breathing, along with activities like mindful walking, can help with our general levels of anxiety.

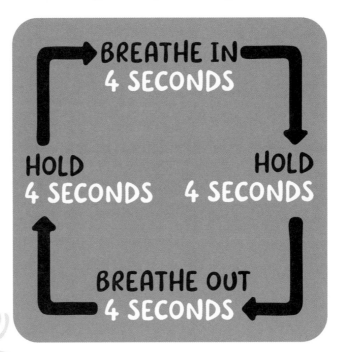

# Brain dump

How are you feeling right now? Sometimes getting our thoughts out onto the page can help us to process and make sense of them.

....................................................................

....................................................................

....................................................................

....................................................................

....................................................................

....................................................................

....................................................................

....................................................................

....................................................................

....................................................................

....................................................................

....................................................................

....................................................................

....................................................................

....................................................................

....................................................................

....................................................................

....................................................................

....................................................................

# How to make a self-soothe box

Self-soothe boxes, also referred to as crisis boxes or sensory boxes, are excellent tools to have access to. They are designed to be full of items that help you to get through periods of distress. Try and fill yours with things that cater to each of your five senses. Here are some suggestions of things you could include that might be helpful:

- ❀ **Taste:** Chocolates or mints, or maybe your favourite teabags

- ❀ **Smell:** Essential oils, nice hand creams or perfume

- ❀ **Touch:** Stress balls, tangles or something soft like a small cuddly toy

- ❀ **Hear:** A prompt card to remind you to access your happy playlist or favourite song

- ❀ **See:** Photos of people you love, motivational quotes or perhaps some letters of encouragement

It might also be helpful to keep a list of enjoyable activities, helplines or apps that you find useful when you are finding things difficult.

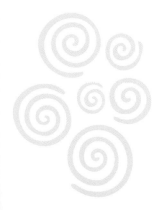

# What will go in my self-soothe box?

.......................................................................................

.......................................................................................

.......................................................................................

.......................................................................................

.......................................................................................

.......................................................................................

.......................................................................................

.......................................................................................

.......................................................................................

.......................................................................................

.......................................................................................

.......................................................................................

.......................................................................................

.......................................................................................

.......................................................................................

.......................................................................................

.......................................................................................

.......................................................................................

.......................................................................................

.......................................................................................

.......................................................................................

.......................................................................................

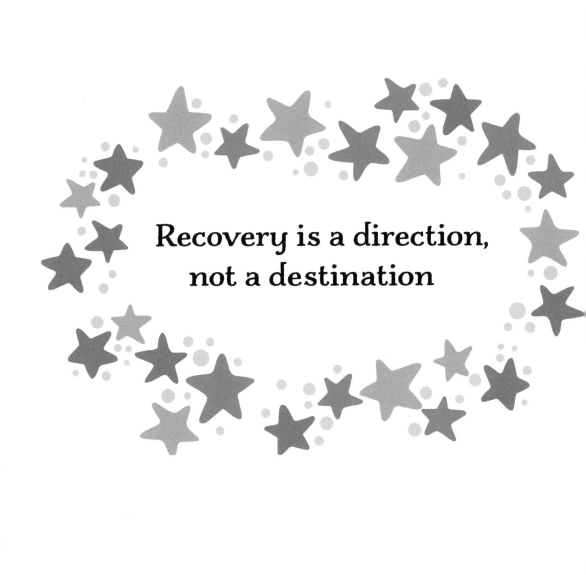

Recovery is a direction,
not a destination

How are you feeling today? Draw or write it out!

# Coping statements

When we are anxious or upset, it can feel like those feelings are going to last forever. Here are some things you can say to yourself to get you through.

**1.** Listen to what your OCD is saying and do the opposite.

**2.** OCD does not keep you safe; recovery keeps you safe.

**3.** Intrusive thoughts do not define you. They do not make you a bad person.

**4.** Make molehills out of a mountain. Approach one thing at a time; they will add up.

**5.** Performing a compulsion is not a failure. It's the effort to resist that counts / Try again next time / Keep going with the fight.

**6.** Acknowledge what you're feeling; sit with it instead of trying to make it disappear. Allowing discomfort to exist in the present helps it decrease in the future.

**7.** Making changes can be scary, but not as scary as staying the same.

**8.** Sometimes the best thing for you is the thing that feels the worst. That feeling is temporary and worth enduring to achieve positive change, even when you can't see it on the horizon.

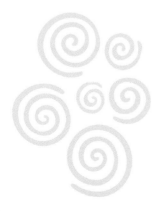

# My skills and strengths

Everybody has their own individual strengths that we can draw upon when things feel difficult. What are some of yours? If you feel stuck, it can help to ask the people around you their thoughts.

1. ........................................................................................
........................................................................................

2. ........................................................................................
........................................................................................

3. ........................................................................................
........................................................................................

4. ........................................................................................
........................................................................................

5. ........................................................................................
........................................................................................

6. ........................................................................................
........................................................................................

7. ........................................................................................
........................................................................................

8. ........................................................................................
........................................................................................

9. ........................................................................................
........................................................................................

10. ........................................................................................
........................................................................................

# What would I say to a friend if they were going through this?

Having an illness like OCD, which can affect many areas of our lives and those around us, can often result in feelings of guilt and shame and we can be harder on ourselves than we need to be. Remember, it's not your fault that you have a mental illness. What would you say to a friend if they were going through something similar?

......................................................................................................

......................................................................................................

......................................................................................................

......................................................................................................

......................................................................................................

......................................................................................................

......................................................................................................

......................................................................................................

......................................................................................................

......................................................................................................

......................................................................................................

......................................................................................................

......................................................................................................

......................................................................................................

......................................................................................................

......................................................................................................

# Recovery prompts

Sometimes we might need reminders to prompt us to stay focused on recovery, especially as some compulsions might feel like they have become part of your day-to-day routine.

Try getting some funky sticky notes and write affirmations on them. Stick them around the house where you struggle most with compulsions or intrusive thoughts. For example: 'I am stronger than my anxiety' next to a light switch or 'This discomfort will pass' on a door.

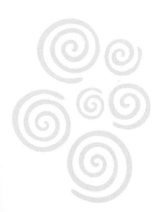

# Why do I want to be well?

Letting go of an illness like OCD can be really challenging, because it takes up so much of our time and brain space, and can also help us to feel safe. Use this space to think about why you would like to get better, and reflect back on it when you feel like you've hit a road block.

# Pros and cons of change

Sometimes, you might feel that you don't want to recover – this is a normal feeling and lots of people will experience it. It can be helpful to weigh up the pros and cons of making recovery focused decisions, as this can help you to reflect on the benefits of making changes.

## What are the pros of recovering?

...............................................................................

...............................................................................

...............................................................................

...............................................................................

...............................................................................

...............................................................................

...............................................................................

## What are the cons of recovering?

...............................................................................

...............................................................................

...............................................................................

...............................................................................

...............................................................................

...............................................................................

...............................................................................

# What are the pros of not recovering?

......................................................................................

......................................................................................

......................................................................................

......................................................................................

......................................................................................

......................................................................................

......................................................................................

# What are the cons of not recovering?

......................................................................................

......................................................................................

......................................................................................

......................................................................................

......................................................................................

......................................................................................

......................................................................................

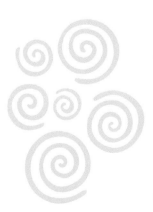

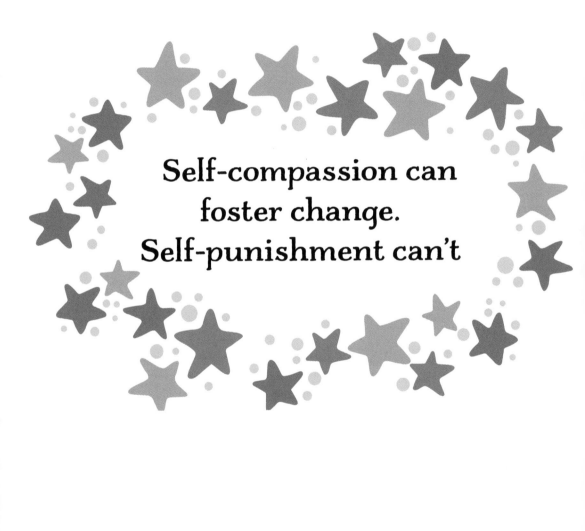

Self-compassion can foster change. Self-punishment can't

# Brain dump

How are you feeling right now? Sometimes getting our thoughts out onto the page can help us to process and make sense of them.

.........................................................................

.........................................................................

.........................................................................

.........................................................................

.........................................................................

.........................................................................

.........................................................................

.........................................................................

.........................................................................

.........................................................................

.........................................................................

.........................................................................

.........................................................................

.........................................................................

.........................................................................

.........................................................................

.........................................................................

.........................................................................

.........................................................................

.........................................................................

.........................................................................

.........................................................................

# People who inspire me

We can draw inspiration from lots of different places, but sometimes having people we look up to can be really helpful. Who inspires you to be your best self?

1. ..................................................................................
..................................................................................

2. ..................................................................................
..................................................................................

3. ..................................................................................
..................................................................................

4. ..................................................................................
..................................................................................

5. ..................................................................................
..................................................................................

6. ..................................................................................
..................................................................................

7. ..................................................................................
..................................................................................

8. ..................................................................................
..................................................................................

9. ..................................................................................
..................................................................................

10. ..................................................................................
..................................................................................

# Positive words wordsearch

The first three words you see are your words of the day.

| W | D | Q | B | O | K | Z | D | F | K | P | R | S | G |
|---|---|---|---|---|---|---|---|---|---|---|---|---|---|
| B | S | H | R | N | B | I | W | A | U | Z | K | H | F |
| K | U | E | I | J | B | U | G | R | K | T | F | S | Z |
| E | B | M | R | O | M | B | A | L | W | C | U | W | E |
| H | B | P | V | P | C | W | H | X | M | A | W | R | L |
| P | X | O | Z | E | E | J | Y | T | Q | F | E | G | E |
| S | B | W | P | O | W | E | R | F | U | L | J | Q | A |
| C | Z | E | G | N | T | O | V | E | R | C | O | M | E |
| N | G | R | O | W | T | H | R | Y | S | S | F | Q | C |
| S | D | E | T | E | R | M | I | N | A | T | I | O | N |
| A | U | D | B | V | U | A | E | H | O | P | E | M | K |
| F | O | R | W | A | R | D | S | N | L | Y | P | F | V |
| F | D | G | F | W | B | F | I | G | H | T | E | R | P |
| R | O | F | R | E | E | D | O | M | H | X | N | D | F |

DETERMINATION    POWERFUL    HOPE

EMPOWERED    FIGHTER    GROWTH

FUTURE    FORWARDS

FREEDOM    OVERCOME

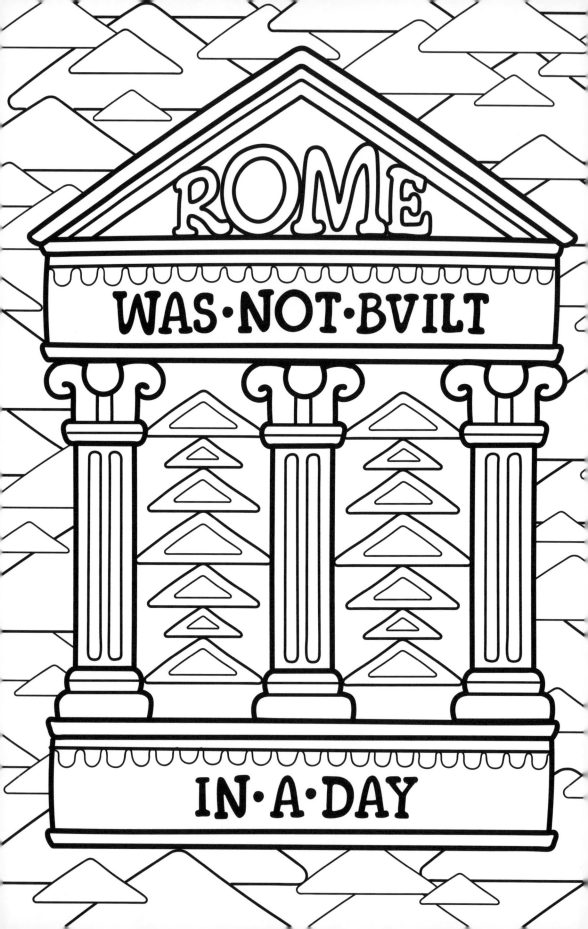

# Letter writing

It can sometimes be helpful to view OCD as something separate from us. What would you say to your OCD if you could?

# What stressful life events increase my OCD symptoms?

There are going to be stressful periods over the course of your life that might make OCD rear its head.

## What sort of events might these be?

..................................................................................................

..................................................................................................

..................................................................................................

..................................................................................................

..................................................................................................

..................................................................................................

..................................................................................................

## What is helpful for me when things feel difficult?

Once we have identified things that increase our OCD symptoms, we can start to notice them more. The world can be a difficult place at times and sometimes we are going to come across things that feel difficult. How can you cope with or manage these experiences?

..................................................................................................

..................................................................................................

..................................................................................................

..................................................................................................

..................................................................................................

..................................................................................................

..................................................................................................

## What do I do currently that decreases my OCD symptoms?

This might include things like connecting with people I love, resisting my compulsions and doing things that scare me.

································································································

································································································

································································································

································································································

································································································

································································································

································································································

## What can I try to do that reduces my symptoms even further?

································································································

································································································

································································································

································································································

································································································

································································································

································································································

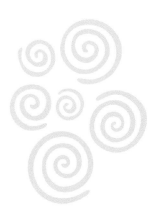

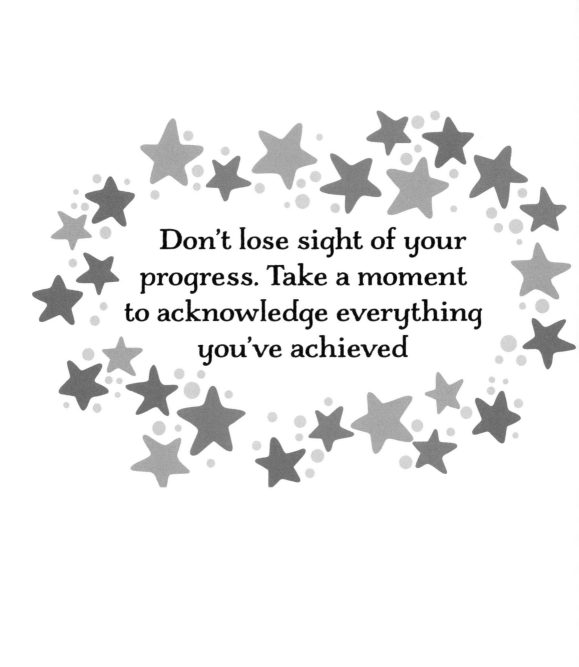

Don't lose sight of your progress. Take a moment to acknowledge everything you've achieved

# How are you feeling today? Draw or write it out!

# OCD tool: facing fears gradually

Part of moving forward with recovery from OCD is gradually facing your fears, whilst resisting compulsions. This is called Exposure and Response Prevention (E/RP). We can do this by creating a hierarchy of OCD compulsions: all the things OCD makes you do, avoid or things others do. Here we will start to put together a ladder of compulsions, starting from the ones that are the easiest to resist, moving up to the ones that are the most difficult. You will then have a go at trying to resist an OCD compulsion by doing the opposite of what OCD wants.

Some examples might be:

❅ Touching something you feel is dirty without washing your hands

❅ Leaving the house without checking the door is locked

❅ Going 15 minutes without doing a frequently occurring compulsion

❅ Touching something with only one side of your body

❅ Only turning off the light switch once

Everybody's experience of OCD is completely unique and you will have your own individual compulsions which we identified earlier, but we hope the above suggestions will act as a prompt to help you to come up with some of your own.

| | E/RP task | Level of anxiety (0–100%) |
|---|---|---|
| 1. | | |
| 2. | | |
| 3. | | |
| 4. | | |
| 5. | | |
| 6. | | |
| 7. | | |
| 8. | | |
| 9. | | |
| 10. | | |

## Why do we do E/RP?

When we experience an obsession our anxiety increases. Completing a compulsion then makes anxiety go down again, so we continue doing this despite the fact the relief is short lived.

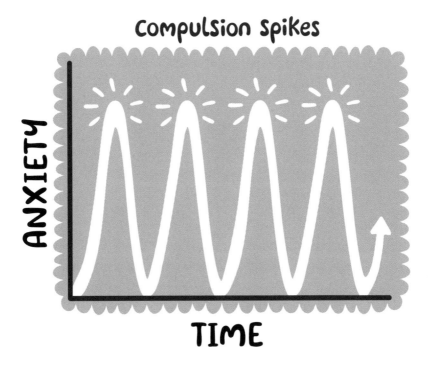

Compulsion Spikes

ANXIETY

TIME

Through doing this, we never get to find out what happens if we don't carry out the compulsion, and whether our anxiety would start to reduce even if we didn't listen to OCD.

If we resist a compulsion, we find that over time our anxiety starts to go down on its own. This is called habituation and means our body is getting used to anxiety. If we keep resisting the compulsion, each time we will find this easier and our anxiety starts to come down more quickly.

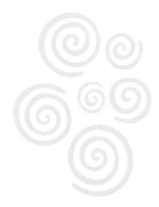

# Steps for practising your first E/RP

1. Pick a compulsion from your OCD hierarchy.

2. What is the obsession or fear this compulsion relates to?

3. What will your exposure be? How can you face the fear?

4. What will the response prevention be? How can you resist the ritual or do the opposite of what OCD wants?

5. Can you do this all in one go or do you need to break it down into steps?

6. How anxious did you feel straight after the task? What about 5, 10, 20 minutes later? Keep rating anxiety over the next hour to see what happens.

7. What happens to your anxiety the more you practise the task?

# OCD tricks to look out for!

❈ Try not to reassure yourself or seek reassurance from others; this is an OCD compulsion.

❈ Try not to distract yourself when practising the E/RP; sit with the feeling of anxiety.

❈ Try to resist mental rituals.

❈ Practise, practise, practise! The more you resist OCD, the easier it becomes.

It might be helpful to start making a list of E/RP tasks you have completed here and add to this as you go, so you can reflect back on your progress and your achievements.

.......................................................................................

.......................................................................................

.......................................................................................

.......................................................................................

......................................................................

......................................................................

......................................................................

......................................................................

......................................................................

......................................................................

......................................................................

......................................................................

## Learning from E/RP

You might now have made some steps to move to the top of your hierarchy. What have you learned since you started carrying out E/RP? What happens to your anxiety over time? Have any compulsions become easier to resist?

......................................................................

......................................................................

......................................................................

......................................................................

......................................................................

......................................................................

......................................................................

......................................................................

......................................................................

......................................................................

......................................................................

# Taking on the scientist role

When completing E/RP tasks, you may find that what happens when you resist an OCD compulsion is not what you expect. OCD makes us overestimate the degree of danger or threat involved with not carrying out compulsions – it can be helpful to think of OCD as a faulty fire alarm that is activating when there is no fire present. Sometimes it can be helpful to reflect on what we thought might happen before challenging our OCD and what actually happens. To do this, you can take the role of a scientist by making predictions and observing what actually happens. As a scientist, in order to make it a fair test, try to resist all compulsions when carrying out a task.

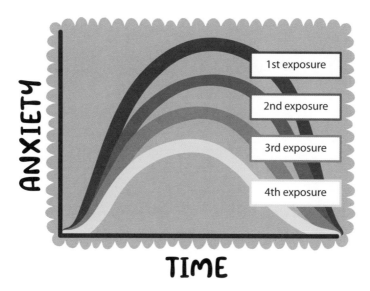

### OCD tricks to look out for!

* Remember we can never be 100% certain about whether something will happen in the future or has happened in the past. Beating OCD is about tolerating uncertainty.

* OCD might tell you 'this time you were lucky...but next time it won't be the same'. To fight back, try to repeat the task as many times as you can.

What am I going to do and for how long?

...........................................................................................................

...........................................................................................................

What do I predict is going to happen?

...........................................................................................................

...........................................................................................................

How strongly do I believe this prediction? (0–100%)

...........................................................................................................

...........................................................................................................

What actually happened?

...........................................................................................................

...........................................................................................................

What did I learn?

...........................................................................................................

...........................................................................................................

How anxious did I feel at the beginning,
at its highest and at the end?

...........................................................................................................

...........................................................................................................

Do I need to repeat the exposure?

...........................................................................................................

...........................................................................................................

Do I need to do anything differently next time?

...........................................................................................................

...........................................................................................................

What am I going to do and for how long?

.......................................................................

.......................................................................

What do I predict is going to happen?

.......................................................................

.......................................................................

How strongly do I believe this prediction? (0–100%)

.......................................................................

.......................................................................

What actually happened?

.......................................................................

.......................................................................

What did I learn?

.......................................................................

.......................................................................

How anxious did I feel at the beginning,
at its highest and at the end?

.......................................................................

.......................................................................

Do I need to repeat the exposure?

.......................................................................

.......................................................................

Do I need to do anything differently next time?

.......................................................................

.......................................................................

What am I going to do and for how long?

.............................................................................

.............................................................................

What do I predict is going to happen?

.............................................................................

.............................................................................

How strongly do I believe this prediction? (0–100%)

.............................................................................

.............................................................................

What actually happened?

.............................................................................

.............................................................................

What did I learn?

.............................................................................

.............................................................................

How anxious did I feel at the beginning,
at its highest and at the end?

.............................................................................

.............................................................................

Do I need to repeat the exposure?

.............................................................................

.............................................................................

Do I need to do anything differently next time?

.............................................................................

.............................................................................

What am I going to do and for how long?

......................................................

......................................................

What do I predict is going to happen?

......................................................

......................................................

How strongly do I believe this prediction? (0–100%)

......................................................

......................................................

What actually happened?

......................................................

......................................................

What did I learn?

......................................................

......................................................

How anxious did I feel at the beginning,
at its highest and at the end?

......................................................

......................................................

Do I need to repeat the exposure?

......................................................

......................................................

Do I need to do anything differently next time?

......................................................

......................................................

What am I going to do and for how long?

.................................................................

.................................................................

What do I predict is going to happen?

.................................................................

.................................................................

How strongly do I believe this prediction? (0–100%)

.................................................................

.................................................................

What actually happened?

.................................................................

.................................................................

What did I learn?

.................................................................

.................................................................

How anxious did I feel at the beginning,
at its highest and at the end?

.................................................................

.................................................................

Do I need to repeat the exposure?

.................................................................

.................................................................

Do I need to do anything differently next time?

.................................................................

.................................................................

What am I going to do and for how long?

.........................................................................

.........................................................................

What do I predict is going to happen?

.........................................................................

.........................................................................

How strongly do I believe this prediction? (0–100%)

.........................................................................

.........................................................................

What actually happened?

.........................................................................

.........................................................................

What did I learn?

.........................................................................

.........................................................................

How anxious did I feel at the beginning,
at its highest and at the end?

.........................................................................

.........................................................................

Do I need to repeat the exposure?

.........................................................................

.........................................................................

Do I need to do anything differently next time?

.........................................................................

.........................................................................

What am I going to do and for how long?

......................................................................

......................................................................

What do I predict is going to happen?

......................................................................

......................................................................

How strongly do I believe this prediction? (0–100%)

......................................................................

......................................................................

What actually happened?

......................................................................

......................................................................

What did I learn?

......................................................................

......................................................................

How anxious did I feel at the beginning,
at its highest and at the end?

......................................................................

......................................................................

Do I need to repeat the exposure?

......................................................................

......................................................................

Do I need to do anything differently next time?

......................................................................

......................................................................

What am I going to do and for how long?

........................................................

........................................................

What do I predict is going to happen?

........................................................

........................................................

How strongly do I believe this prediction? (0–100%)

........................................................

........................................................

What actually happened?

........................................................

........................................................

What did I learn?

........................................................

........................................................

How anxious did I feel at the beginning,
at its highest and at the end?

........................................................

........................................................

Do I need to repeat the exposure?

........................................................

........................................................

Do I need to do anything differently next time?

........................................................

........................................................

What am I going to do and for how long?

..................................................................

..................................................................

What do I predict is going to happen?

..................................................................

..................................................................

How strongly do I believe this prediction? (0–100%)

..................................................................

..................................................................

What actually happened?

..................................................................

..................................................................

What did I learn?

..................................................................

..................................................................

How anxious did I feel at the beginning,
at its highest and at the end?

..................................................................

..................................................................

Do I need to repeat the exposure?

..................................................................

..................................................................

Do I need to do anything differently next time?

..................................................................

..................................................................

What am I going to do and for how long?

..........................................................................

..........................................................................

What do I predict is going to happen?

..........................................................................

..........................................................................

How strongly do I believe this prediction? (0–100%)

..........................................................................

..........................................................................

What actually happened?

..........................................................................

..........................................................................

What did I learn?

..........................................................................

..........................................................................

How anxious did I feel at the beginning,
at its highest and at the end?

..........................................................................

..........................................................................

Do I need to repeat the exposure?

..........................................................................

..........................................................................

Do I need to do anything differently next time?

..........................................................................

..........................................................................

# How are you feeling today? Draw or write it out!

# Recovery jar

It can sometimes be difficult to think of reasons and strategies to challenge your OCD in the moment, especially if you're feeling anxious or overwhelmed. Try taking a clean jar and fill it with notes of ways you can challenge your OCD. Pick a note out of the jar on a consistent regular basis and face that challenge. This can help maintain consistency and keep you making continuous progress.

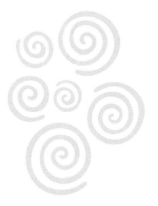

# Early warning signs

It is possible to make a full and sustained recovery from OCD; however, people can often be vulnerable to lapses or relapses in times of stress or uncertainty. What are some early warning signs that things are getting more difficult which you and the people around you should be aware of?

..................................................................................

..................................................................................

..................................................................................

..................................................................................

..................................................................................

..................................................................................

..................................................................................

..................................................................................

..................................................................................

..................................................................................

..................................................................................

..................................................................................

..................................................................................

..................................................................................

..................................................................................

..................................................................................

..................................................................................

..................................................................................

# My traffic lights

Sometimes it can be helpful to think of our progress in terms of a traffic light system: red meaning relapse, we are noticing a lot of distressing, intrusive thoughts and we are spending a lot of time and energy on compulsions, orange meaning we are noticing some OCD compulsions creeping in and need to try to do the opposite of what OCD wants, and green meaning we are staying well from OCD, are able to let our unpleasant thoughts go and are resisting the urge to carry out rituals. Have a think about what life looks like for you in each of these zones and what your plan of action would be for each one.

## What does my green zone look like?

..................................................................................

..................................................................................

..................................................................................

..................................................................................

..................................................................................

..................................................................................

## How can I stay in this zone?

..................................................................................

..................................................................................

..................................................................................

..................................................................................

..................................................................................

..................................................................................

## What does my orange zone look like?

. . . . . . . . . . . . . . . . . . . . . . . . . . . . . . . . . . . . . . . . . . . . . . . . . . . . . . . . . .

. . . . . . . . . . . . . . . . . . . . . . . . . . . . . . . . . . . . . . . . . . . . . . . . . . . . . . . . . .

. . . . . . . . . . . . . . . . . . . . . . . . . . . . . . . . . . . . . . . . . . . . . . . . . . . . . . . . . .

. . . . . . . . . . . . . . . . . . . . . . . . . . . . . . . . . . . . . . . . . . . . . . . . . . . . . . . . . .

. . . . . . . . . . . . . . . . . . . . . . . . . . . . . . . . . . . . . . . . . . . . . . . . . . . . . . . . . .

. . . . . . . . . . . . . . . . . . . . . . . . . . . . . . . . . . . . . . . . . . . . . . . . . . . . . . . . . .

## How can I get out of this zone?

. . . . . . . . . . . . . . . . . . . . . . . . . . . . . . . . . . . . . . . . . . . . . . . . . . . . . . . . . .

. . . . . . . . . . . . . . . . . . . . . . . . . . . . . . . . . . . . . . . . . . . . . . . . . . . . . . . . . .

. . . . . . . . . . . . . . . . . . . . . . . . . . . . . . . . . . . . . . . . . . . . . . . . . . . . . . . . . .

. . . . . . . . . . . . . . . . . . . . . . . . . . . . . . . . . . . . . . . . . . . . . . . . . . . . . . . . . .

. . . . . . . . . . . . . . . . . . . . . . . . . . . . . . . . . . . . . . . . . . . . . . . . . . . . . . . . . .

. . . . . . . . . . . . . . . . . . . . . . . . . . . . . . . . . . . . . . . . . . . . . . . . . . . . . . . . . .

## What does my red zone look like?

. . . . . . . . . . . . . . . . . . . . . . . . . . . . . . . . . . . . . . . . . . . . . . . . . . . . . . . . . .

. . . . . . . . . . . . . . . . . . . . . . . . . . . . . . . . . . . . . . . . . . . . . . . . . . . . . . . . . .

. . . . . . . . . . . . . . . . . . . . . . . . . . . . . . . . . . . . . . . . . . . . . . . . . . . . . . . . . .

. . . . . . . . . . . . . . . . . . . . . . . . . . . . . . . . . . . . . . . . . . . . . . . . . . . . . . . . . .

. . . . . . . . . . . . . . . . . . . . . . . . . . . . . . . . . . . . . . . . . . . . . . . . . . . . . . . . . .

. . . . . . . . . . . . . . . . . . . . . . . . . . . . . . . . . . . . . . . . . . . . . . . . . . . . . . . . . .

## How can I get out of this zone?

........................................................................................

........................................................................................

........................................................................................

........................................................................................

........................................................................................

........................................................................................

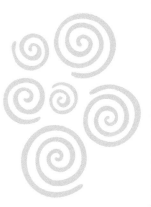

# Brain dump

How are you feeling right now? Sometimes getting our thoughts out onto the page can help us to process and make sense of them.

.......................................................................................................

.......................................................................................................

.......................................................................................................

.......................................................................................................

.......................................................................................................

.......................................................................................................

.......................................................................................................

.......................................................................................................

.......................................................................................................

.......................................................................................................

.......................................................................................................

.......................................................................................................

.......................................................................................................

.......................................................................................................

.......................................................................................................

.......................................................................................................

.......................................................................................................

.......................................................................................................

.......................................................................................................

.......................................................................................................

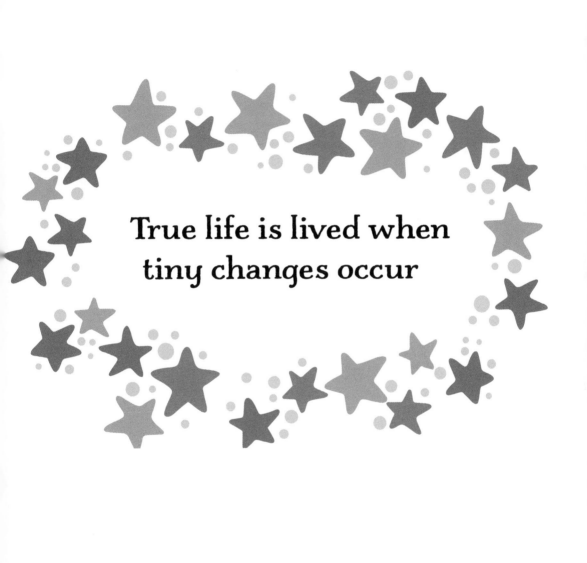

True life is lived when
tiny changes occur

# Managing setbacks

It's important to not only notice when things are starting to get difficult, but also to plan for what situations might result in this happening. What do you think could cause a potential lapse or relapse for you?

## What could cause a setback?

.......................................................................................
.......................................................................................
.......................................................................................
.......................................................................................
.......................................................................................
.......................................................................................
.......................................................................................
.......................................................................................

## How could I manage this?

.......................................................................................
.......................................................................................
.......................................................................................
.......................................................................................
.......................................................................................
.......................................................................................
.......................................................................................
.......................................................................................

# Keeping well

There are lots of things we need to do to keep ourselves on track, some every day and some less often. Have a think about what some of these are for you.

### What can I do on a daily basis to keep myself well?

........................................................................................

........................................................................................

........................................................................................

........................................................................................

........................................................................................

........................................................................................

........................................................................................

........................................................................................

### What can I do on a weekly basis to keep myself well?

........................................................................................

........................................................................................

........................................................................................

........................................................................................

........................................................................................

........................................................................................

........................................................................................

........................................................................................

# What do I need to do less often to keep myself well?

.........................................................................................

.........................................................................................

.........................................................................................

.........................................................................................

.........................................................................................

.........................................................................................

.........................................................................................

.........................................................................................

# How are you feeling today? Draw or write it out!

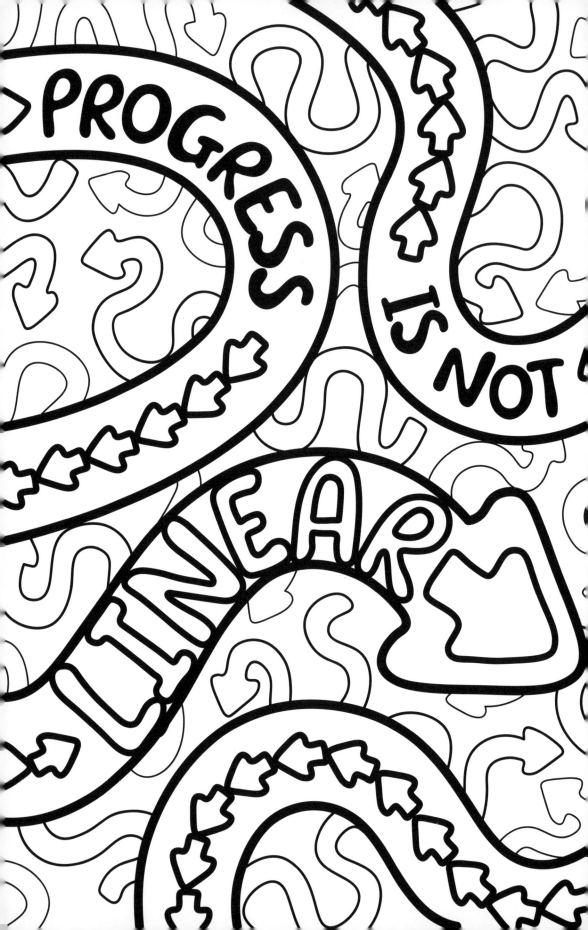

# What have I achieved since starting this journal?

We hope that over the time you have been working through this book you have been able to start thinking more about ways you can manage and overcome your OCD. What are some of the things you have achieved, no matter how big or small, since you started using this journal?

........................................................................

........................................................................

........................................................................

........................................................................

........................................................................

........................................................................

........................................................................

........................................................................

........................................................................

........................................................................

........................................................................

........................................................................

........................................................................

........................................................................

........................................................................

........................................................................

........................................................................

........................................................................

Congratulations, reader!

You've worked your way through this journal. We hope that you have found some of these exercises useful and that they have got you thinking about ways you can challenge your OCD, and start building a life without it.

There are ways you can continue seeking support, which you will find in the back of this book – these have been recommended by Phoebe as resources that have been helpful for them in their own recovery.

We wish you all the luck in the world for your life beyond this journal. Remember, you are more than just your illness. Be kind to yourself.

Lots of love, Cara and Phoebe

# Useful Resources

## Websites

OCD Action: www.ocdaction.org.uk

OCD UK: www.ocduk.org

International OCD Foundation: www.iocdf.org

## Books

Challacombe, F., Bream Oldfield, V. and Salkovskis, P. M. (2011) *Break Free from OCD: Overcoming Obsessive Compulsive Disorder with CBT*. London: Vermillion.

Derisley, J., Heyman, I., Robinson, S. and Turner, C. (2008) *Breaking Free from OCD: A CBT Guide for Young People and Their Families*. London: Jessica Kingsley Publishers.

Greenberger, D. and Padesky, C. A. (2016) *Mind Over Mood: Change How You Feel by Changing the Way You Think*. New York: The Guilford Press.

Mazza, M. T. (2020) *The ACT Workbook for OCD: Mindfulness, Acceptance, and Exposure Skills to Live Well with Obsessive-Compulsive Disorder*. Oakland: New Harbinger Publications.

# Acknowledgements

## Cara

I am grateful to my family and friends who are always so supportive of my writing projects. I am especially grateful to Phoebe, whose contributions have enriched and added endless value to this book.

However, the people I owe the most thanks to are my clients who, despite unimaginable difficulties, show up to therapy and teach me something new every time. It is an honour and a privilege to get to support people struggling with what can be an incredibly cruel and isolating illness, and the experience of walking alongside people who are brave enough to challenge themselves in the face of such anxiety is something I do not take for granted.

A massive thank you also goes to Dr Hannah Baker, who kindly shared her expertise and experience when supporting us to create the best resource we could for people living with OCD.

I hope that I have been able to use all I have learned from working with people with OCD and created a resource that will be helpful for readers at whatever stage of their journey they are at.

## Phoebe

Thank you Cara for inviting me to contribute to this book; it's always an honour when my lived experience is recognized as expertise in its own right.

Much like Cara, thank you to the people I have supported as peer support worker in the NHS, and my colleagues who have endless faith in what I contribute to our service. This job, and by extension the people I have met doing it, has solidified my recovery and changed my professional and personal trajectory.

Weirdly, thank you to OCD. As much suffering as it has caused, I wouldn't be where I am in life without it. It ultimately has led me to my passion to create change. I can't imagine who I'd be if I hadn't developed OCD all those years ago.

# About the Authors

Cara Lisette has struggled with mental illness for much of her life, and through these experiences discovered her love of journalling. She has always seen the value in creativity in fostering good mental health and this has been endlessly helpful in her own journey towards recovery.

Cara is a registered mental health nurse and qualified psychological therapist. She also runs a successful blog about mental health (www.caras-corner.com) and is active on twitter (@caralisette) and Instagram (@caralisette), where she talks about her own mental health and recovery in addition to sharing tips and knowledge about mental health overall, from both her personal and professional experiences. She is the author of *The Eating Disorder Recovery Journal* and *The Bipolar Journal*, which are based on her knowledge as a therapist and her lived experience of mental illness.

Phoebe Webb is a campaigner for better awareness and treatment of mental illness, inspired by her ongoing recovery from anorexia nervosa and obsessive-compulsive disorder as a late-diagnosed autistic queer person. Over the years she has contributed to major publications, including *i Newspaper*, *Cosmopolitan* and ITV News, talking about her lived experience of mental health issues. Since 2021 Phoebe has been working as a peer support worker in the NHS, inspiring hope for mental health recovery by working directly with adults in an acute psychiatric hospital, and teenagers with eating disorders in the community. Adoring working in this field, Phoebe is now training as an integrative psychotherapist, believing that lived experience is key in improving mental health services. Additionally, she hosts her own podcast *Not About Food*, exploring the intersectionality of eating disorders. You can follow her activism and find out about her own recovery process on Twitter (@feehlo) and by listening to *Not About Food* wherever you stream podcasts.

*Discover more books from this series...*

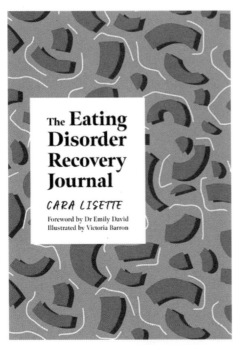

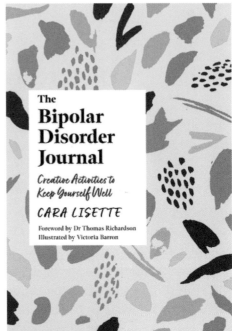

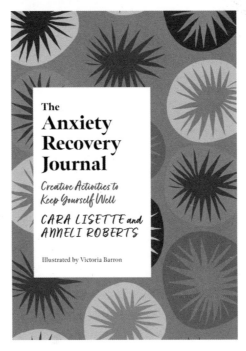